Strength Training Secrets

Build Muscle and Burn Fat

By

Oscar Hammond

Before this document is duplicated or recreated in any form, the consent of the publisher must be obtained.

So therefore, the contents therein cannot be stored electronically, transferred or stored in a database. In no account should the document be copied, scanned, faxed, or retained in whole or in part without the publisher or creator's consent.

Table of Contents

Introduction

In a world where health and fitness have become buzzwords, and the pursuit of a perfect physique often appears perplexing, there is a secret treasure trove of knowledge just waiting to be discovered. Welcome to "Strength Training Secrets: Build Muscle and Burn Fat," a voyage that promises not just physical transformation but also a profound shift in perspective, intertwined with my own personal odyssey.

Like many others, I was once lost in a maze of fad diets and fleeting fitness routines, searching for the elusive keys to a stronger, leaner, and healthier self. I fought the scales, battled self-doubt, and almost resigned to the notion that my fitness ambitions were a distant illusion. In these moments of struggle and self-discovery, I discovered the fundamental core of strength training.

My narrative isn't about a natural-born athlete or a fitness expert; it's about the transformational power of determination and education. It was a cool fall morning when I first entered a gym, which would quickly become my sanctuary. I was afraid, a little disoriented, and adamant about changing my life. I had no idea that this seemingly insignificant action would set the stage for an extraordinary trip.

This book is more than just a collection of exercises and dietary advice; it's a road map to comprehending the profound effects of strength training on both the body and the mind. It's a story about the secrets I discovered on my journey, secrets that extend beyond the gym and into the domain of holistic wellness. I learned the keys to not just growing muscle and burning fat, but also cultivating a tough, confident, and disciplined mindset, via sweat, perseverance, and numerous hours of research.

We will delve into the principles of strength training, decipher the mysteries of nutrition, and investigate the art of creating a personalized workout plan as we progress through the chapters of this book. You will gain knowledge of advanced tactics, discover how to overcome plateaus and find the determination to push yourself beyond your boundaries. This journey, however, is about more than just physical transformation; it is about harnessing the power inside, linking the mind and body, and setting out on a path to long-term health and wellness.

My aim is that my narrative will inspire you. "Strength Training Secrets" has something for everyone, whether you are a beginner looking to get started or a seasoned fitness enthusiast looking to fine-tune your technique.

So, let us go on this life-changing trip together. Prepare to discover your latent potential, sculpt your body, and ignite a newfound passion for health and fitness. As I reveal the secrets that changed my life, I ask you to find the immense strength that is waiting to be released within you.

Are you willing to get involved? I know your answer will be a yes!

Let's delve into the secrets that will assist you in building muscle, burning fat, and embarking on a life-changing experience.

Chapter One

Strength Training Fundamentals

Resistance training is a cornerstone of exercise that has endured the test of time in the world of fitness, where various trends and workouts come and go like transient fads. I've gone on a transforming path that has not only transformed my physique but also dramatically reshaped my life. In this first chapter, let's dig deep into the realm of resistance training, delving into its fundamentals, advantages, and incredible narrative of how it became my route to strength and vitality.

Like many others, my personal journey into the world of resistance training began with a desire for change. I'd spent years battling the bulge, hopping from one trendy diet to the next, and chasing distant fitness objectives that seemed to fade further away with each try. I didn't actually begin to improve my body and my life until I discovered the powerful influence of resistance training.

Resistance training, at its most basic, includes the use of external resistance – often weights or resistance bands – to increase strength and muscle hypertrophy. It's a basic but extremely effective idea. The theory behind it is based on the idea of progressive overload, which states that muscles adapt and grow stronger as resistance steadily increases.

The physical advantages of resistance exercise are nothing short of amazing. It's not just about chiseled abs and huge biceps; it's about functional strength that translates into better daily living. Resistance exercise, from greater bone density to improved metabolism, provides the groundwork for a healthier, more vibrant lifestyle.

What actually distinguishes resistance exercise is its effect on the psyche. It is not only about lifting weights; it is also about increasing one's self-esteem and confidence. As my training developed, I discovered an inner resilience I had never known existed. The discipline, drive, and sense of accomplishment that each session provided spilled over into other parts of my life, making me more confident and capable.

Creating an efficient resistance training routine is an art as much as a science. It entails selecting the appropriate exercises, calculating the appropriate number of sets and repetitions, and ensuring adequate recuperation between workouts. My own journey involved trial and error as I fine-tuned my regimen to fit my goals and constraints.

While lifting weights is an important part of resistance training, eating is equally important. I discovered the significance of providing my body with the proper nutrition to assist muscular growth and repair. The combination of a healthy diet and resistance training is the key to realizing its full potential.

Resistance training is not without its difficulties. Plateaus can be discouraging, and injuries are a risk. However, these disappointments might serve as excellent learning opportunities. I discuss my own experiences with plateaus and failures, offering advice on how to overcome them and emerge stronger.

The sense of fellowship that developed with resistance training was one of the most inspiring components of my trip. Whether in the gym or connecting with fellow enthusiasts online, the camaraderie and support were important in terms of staying motivated and accountable.

Common Myths Dispelled

Myths and misconceptions abound in the fitness field, causing barriers to implementing effective and useful workout programs. Resistance training, a foundational component of physical fitness, is not immune to such misconceptions. These fallacies, which are frequently founded on misinformation or outdated beliefs, might discourage people from realizing the myriad benefits that resistance training has to offer. Below, we will deconstruct some of the most common resistance training myths and expose the reality that refutes them.

Myth 1: Lifting Weights Equals Bulkiness

One persistent fallacy holds that resistance training will ultimately result in a bulky, overly muscular appearance. This belief, however, is largely erroneous. Building significant muscular mass in the manner of bodybuilders necessitates specialized training programs, strong dedication, and, in many cases, specific diets or supplements. Resistance training, rather than extreme muscularity, benefits lean muscle development, increased metabolism, and a toned appearance in the normal person.

Myth 2: Age and Fitness Level Matter

Another widely held misunderstanding is that resistance training is only appropriate for the young and physically fit. In actuality, resistance training is appropriate for people of all ages and fitness levels. Whether you're a novice or a seasoned athlete, the routines may be adapted to your talents and goals. Individuals at various phases of life and fitness can benefit from resistance training because of its inclusion.

Myth 3: Danger and Injury

Individuals may be discouraged from participating in resistance training due to concerns about injuries and mishaps. While all physical activities contain some level of risk, resistance training can be risk-free when done appropriately and under adequate supervision. Learning and practicing appropriate form, cautiously increasing weights, and providing adequate recovery time can all help to reduce the probability of injury. In fact, resistance exercise can help avoid injuries by strengthening muscles and improving joint stability.

Myth 4: Cardio Outperforms Resistance in Weight Loss

Another widely held misconception puts cardio against resistance training for weight loss. While cardio exercise burns calories, resistance training has particular advantages for long-term weight management. Resistance exercise resulted in an increase in resting metabolic rate, which leads to continuous calorie expenditure even when resting. Furthermore, regardless of significant weight loss on the scale, the change in body composition achieved with resistance exercise can generate a slimmer appearance.

Myth 5: Expensive Gym Memberships and Equipment are Required

Resistance training is frequently misunderstood as requiring pricey gym memberships or complicated equipment. In truth, effective resistance training can be achieved with little equipment, if any at all, or simply with your own body weight. Resistance bands or dumbbells, along with bodyweight workouts, can produce significant results. Resistance training is no longer limited to individuals with access to specialist gym facilities because of this accessibility.

Myth 6: Women Should Avoid Lifting Heavy Weights

A particularly incorrect belief is directed at women, who are advised to avoid intensive weightlifting for fear of having an overly muscular appearance. Contrary to popular assumption, resistance training, including heavy weight lifting, is beneficial to women's health and well-being. It helps to maintain bone density, improve muscle tone, and promote general strength and functionality. Women can reap various health benefits from resistance training without sacrificing their desired figure.

Warm-up and Safety Precautions

Resistance training is a solid pillar in the realm of fitness, providing individuals with the opportunity to sculpt their bodies and improve their physical and emotional well-being. However, it is not without risk. The trip into the world of weightlifting frequently begins with fervor and ambition, but if not addressed with caution, can result in injuries that impede progress and even put an end to fitness aspirations.

My own foray into resistance training began as a personal change quest. The appeal of building power and muscle, as well as the transformative potential of resistance training, drew me in. However, it didn't take long for me to learn that this adventure needed more than just passion; it demanded a thorough awareness of safety considerations and the significance of adequate warm-up.

Resistance training, like any other physical activity, carries risks. Injuries like strains, sprains, and more severe muscular injuries can occur when workouts are performed incorrectly or without necessary protection. Furthermore, weariness from pushing oneself too hard without enough rest and recovery might lead to accidents.

Adherence to safety procedures is critical for mitigating these hazards and establishing a safe training environment. These precautions include a wide range of issues, from proper form and technique to the use of appropriate equipment. The importance of proper form cannot be emphasized. My own experience has shown me that taking the time to learn the proper manner to perform workouts and continuously prioritizing form minimizes the probability of injury greatly. Using a spotter when lifting big weights is another important safety precaution, providing both physical help and peace of mind during difficult lifts.

However, safety precautions do not stop with form and spotters. The warm-up routine is critical in injury prevention. A well-structured warm-up regimen serves as a barrier against injuries. It prepares the body for physical exertion by gradually boosting heart rate, circulation, and body temperature. It prepares the muscles, making them more supple and resistant to stresses and injuries.

There are numerous components to a successful warm-up. Begin with simple aerobic workouts like jogging or cycling to increase heart rate and circulation, preparing the cardiovascular system for the rigors of resistance training. Following that comes dynamic stretching, which consists of controlled motions that target the muscles that will be used during resistance training. My personal experiences have demonstrated the importance of dynamic stretching; it not only minimizes the risk of injury but also improves overall flexibility and mobility. Another epiphany from my journey was the incorporation of mobility exercises that focus on joint range of motion. These exercises improved joint stability and reduced the likelihood of strains during resistance training.

However, the warm-up ritual is more than just physical preparation. Mental preparation is also essential. Visualization and mental focus are important components of the warm-up phase since they set the tone for a good training session. As my resistance training adventure developed, I learned that psychologically preparing, by visualizing good lifts and being focused, had a direct impact on my performance and safety.

As I continue on my fitness path, I am reminded of the critical need for safety procedures and the warm-up routine. They are more than just a routine; they are a tribute to the wisdom of prioritizing safety and the realization that, when approached with caution, resistance training can be a transforming and injury-free experience.

Chapter Two

Nutrition for Losing Fat and Building Muscle

The significance of pre-workout nutrition in the field of fitness and exercise cannot be understated. It acts as the cornerstone on which your physical performance is built, affecting both your capacity to push through a workout and the efficiency with which your training will help you reach your fitness objectives. The importance of comprehending the nuances of pre-workout nutrition cannot be overstated, whether you are an experienced athlete or a beginner starting your fitness path. This in-depth investigation will cover the crucial elements of pre-workout nutrition, how it affects performance and useful tips for maximizing your pre-workout feed.

Pre-Workout Nutrition

Pre-Workout Nutrition's Function

The main goal of a pre-workout diet is to get your body ready for the physical demands of activity. It accomplishes a number of crucial tasks:

Energy Supply: Pre-workout nutrition's main objective is to give your body the energy it requires to function at its peak. Your muscles need fuel in the form of carbohydrates and lipids to power through an exercise session.

Water: An essential component of a pre-workout diet is enough water. Dehydration can impair performance, cause cramps in the muscles, and raise the risk of injury. You may make sure you're well hydrated before an exercise by drinking enough fluids.

Protein to Support Muscle Growth and Repair: Including a source of protein in your pre-workout diet helps support the maintenance and expansion of your muscles. Protein can be beneficial for long-lasting or strenuous activities, even if carbs are the primary emphasis of pre-workout nutrition.

Important Pre-Workout Nutritional Elements

Let's now examine the essential elements of pre-workout nutrition:

1. Carbohydrates: Your body uses carbohydrates as its main source of energy when you workout. Consuming carbs before exercise helps your muscles and liver restore their glycogen stores, which can reduce tiredness and increase endurance. Choose complex carbs, which provide long-lasting energy, such as whole grains, fruits, and vegetables.

2. Protein: Consuming a small amount of protein before working out can aid in stopping the breakdown of muscles. Lean meats, yogurt, and plant-based protein sources are a few good choices.

3. Fats: While not the main source of energy when exercising, fats can nevertheless offer a steady stream of energy, particularly during

extended activities. Avocados, almonds, and seeds are good sources of healthy fat.

4. Hydration: For best results, proper hydration is essential. While electrolyte drinks can help you restore lost salt, potassium, and other vital minerals during longer or more strenuous workouts, water is still necessary.

5. Timing: A crucial component of pre-workout nutrition is timing. Your pre-exercise meal or snack should ideally be had one to three hours prior to your workout. This provides ample time for your body to consume and assimilate the nutrients.

6. Supplements: A few people choose to take supplements as part of their pre-workout routine. Caffeine, which boosts energy and alertness, and branched-chain amino acids (BCAAs), which assist muscles, are popular pre-workout supplements. However, it's crucial to utilize supplements responsibly and seek medical advice as necessary.

Realistic Pre-Workout Nutrition Techniques

The following are some doable tips for maximizing your pre-workout nutrition:

Balanced Meal: Aim for a meal that is balanced by including carbohydrates, protein, and fats. An ideal pre-workout meal might be, for instance, a whole-grain sandwich with turkey and avocado and a side of fruit.

Simple Snacks: If you're short on time, a quick snack will do. A rapid energy boost can be obtained from foods like a banana with peanut butter or Greek yogurt with berries.

Keep Hydrated: Stay hydrated all day long, especially if you have an afternoon or nighttime workout scheduled.

Experiment and Listen to Your Body: There is no one-size-fits-all pre-workout nutrition, so experiment and pay attention to your body. To determine what is ideal for your body and your workouts, experiment with different diets and times of day.

Avoid Overeating: While it's necessary to nourish your body, you should try to avoid eating large, filling meals just before a workout because they might make you feel uncomfortable and lethargic.

Use Supplements Wisely: If you decide to take supplements, be sure to use them as directed and in the suggested dosages. Keep in mind that dietary supplements cannot replace a balanced diet.

Post-Workout Nutrition

The Function of Post-Exercise Nutrition

Post-workout nutrition fulfills a number of essential roles:

Muscle Recovery: Your muscles are stressed and damaged after exercise, particularly resistance training. After-workout nourishment gives the body the nutrients it needs to rebuild and repair muscular tissues.

Refilling Glycogen Reserves: When you exercise, your body uses stored glycogen (carbohydrates) as fuel. Refueling with carbohydrates after exercise helps you recuperate and become ready for the next workout.

Protein Synthesis: Consuming protein after working out encourages the process through which your body creates new muscle tissue. For the growth and healing of muscles, this is essential.

Hydration: Adequate hydration after exercise aids in replenishing fluids lost through perspiration and supports a number of body processes, such as circulation and nutrient delivery.

Important Post-Workout Nutrition Elements

Let's now examine the essential elements of post-workout nutrition:

1. Protein: Protein is essential for muscle growth and repair. The amino acids required for these activities are provided by protein consumption after exercise. Lean meats, chicken, fish, dairy products, eggs, plant-based choices like tofu and legumes, and protein supplements like whey or plant-based protein powder are all excellent sources of protein.

2. Carbs: The replenishment of glycogen reserves depends on carbohydrates. Sources of high-quality carbohydrates include fruits, vegetables, and whole grains. Particularly after strenuous exercises, simple carbs like fruits might help with a rapid glycogen refill.

3. Hydration: Rehydrating after an exercise is essential to replenish lost fluids and electrolytes. Water is necessary, but for longer or more severe workouts, think about switching to an electrolyte drink or sports drink.

4. Timing: The moment you eat or snack after working out is crucial. When your body is most sensitive to nutritional uptake, which is between 30 minutes and 2 hours after your workout, you should try to eat it at this time.

5. Supplements: To hasten healing and muscle rebuilding, some people choose post-workout supplements like branched-chain amino acids (BCAAs) or protein drinks. While these may be advantageous, the core of your post-workout nutrition should still consist of healthy foods.

Realistic Post-Workout Nutrition Techniques

The following are some doable tips for enhancing your post-workout nutrition:

Balanced Meals: Ensure that your lunch contains a balance of protein, carbohydrates, and veggies if your workout and mealtime are the same.

For a balanced post-workout lunch, try quinoa, grilled chicken, and steamed vegetables.

Quick Snacks: Choose a post-workout snack if you don't have time for a complete dinner. Convenient choices include protein shakes with bananas, peanut butter and banana sandwiches, and Greek yogurt with berries.

Protein Timing: While immediate post-workout nutrition is important, it's also helpful to keep including protein in your future meals to encourage more thorough muscle healing and development.

Don't Forget to Hydrate: Prioritize your post-workout nutrition and hydration together. Water should always be your first choice, but if you've perspired a lot throughout your workout, you might want to add a hydrating beverage.

Individualize Your Approach: Everybody has different dietary requirements and preferences. To find out what suits your body and your fitness objectives the best, experiment with different foods and meal times.

Listen to Your Body: Pay attention to how your body reacts to various post-workout nutrition techniques by keeping a close eye on it. Your method should be modified in accordance with your degree of energy, recovery time, and soreness.

Meal Timing Techniques

Meal timing is a choreographer in the complex dance of nutrition who has a big say in how well your body works. Understanding when and how often you eat can affect your energy levels, metabolism, and general health in addition to the conventional three meals a day. We will delve into the subject of meal timing tactics in this thorough investigation, exposing the science behind them and offering helpful advice to help you nourish your body precisely.

Timing Your Meals Scientifically

It's important to align your eating habits with your body's natural rhythms and nutritional requirements when it comes to mealtime. The following fundamental ideas form the basis of the science underpinning meal timing:

Circadian Rhythms: Your body runs on a 24-hour circadian clock that controls a number of physiological functions. Hormone secretion, digestion, and metabolism are some of these processes. Your overall health may be improved by timing your meals with your body's circadian clock.

Hormonal Reaction: The time of your meals affects the release of hormones like leptin and ghrelin, which govern appetite, as well as insulin, which controls blood sugar levels. You can maximize hormonal responses to aid in weight management and energy balance by carefully planning the timing of your meals.

Nutrient Partitioning: Your body distributes the calories from your meals according to the concept of nutrient partitioning. For instance, eating carbs after working out can encourage the replenishment of muscle glycogen, whereas eating meals high in protein can encourage the synthesis of muscle protein.

Meal Timing Techniques

Intermittent Fasting: Alternating between eating and fasting times is known as intermittent fasting. The 5:2 strategy (five days of regular eating and two days of very reduced calorie intake) and the 16/8 method (16 hours of fasting followed by an 8-hour eating window) are popular approaches. Blood sugar regulation, metabolic health, and weight management can all be improved by intermittent fasting.

Time-Restricted Eating: Time-restricted eating limits the number of hours you can eat each day. You might, for instance, consume all of your meals during a 10-hour period. This method, which synchronizes meal time with circadian rhythms, can be particularly helpful for managing weight.

Nutrition Before and After Exercise: Planning your meals around your workouts will maximize energy and recovery. Before exercising, eat a balanced breakfast or snack with carbohydrates and protein to give your muscles fuel and support their performance. A protein and carbohydrate-rich post-workout diet promotes muscle repair and glycogen refueling.

Front-loading Calories: Based on my own perspective, eating more calories in the morning and evening may help with weight management and metabolic health. The use of this strategy can assist in managing hunger and lessen late-night eating because it is in sync with circadian rhythms.

Regular Meal Timing: It's important to be consistent with meal times. Regular mealtimes aid in controlling hunger and preserving stable blood sugar levels. Regular eating habits can interfere with circadian cycles and increase the risk of overeating.

Practical Advice for Timing Meals

Plan Ahead: Create a meal plan that fits with your daily schedule in advance. Your circadian rhythms must be optimized, which requires consistency.

Listen to Your Body: Eat when you're naturally hungry and pay heed to your body's hunger cues. Avoid forcing yourself to adhere to strict eating habits that conflict with your body's necessities.

Prioritize Nutrient Density: Whenever you eat, pay attention to foods that are high in nutrients and contain all the vitamins and minerals your body needs.

Hydrate: Keep yourself hydrated all day long. Sometimes hunger is confused for dehydration.

Consult a Professional: To create a customized meal timing strategy, think about speaking with a registered dietitian or healthcare practitioner if you have specific health objectives or medical concerns.

Chapter Three

Developing a Strength Training Program

A road we take to accomplish our physical and emotional well-being is called a fitness journey. It starts with a beginning place, an awareness of where you are right now, just like any journey. It takes a comprehensive assessment of your body's capabilities, endurance, and general health to determine your present fitness level; it goes beyond looking at numbers on a scale or your capacity to lift a certain amount of weight. I'll discuss the value of determining your current level of fitness while also sharing my own experience in the process.

When I made the decision to start a fitness journey, I realized how important it was to know where I stood in terms of my physical health. It was the result of a long process that started with a desire for change and a higher standard of living. Getting rid of any preconceived ideas I had about what being "fit" meant was my first step. It was about achieving a condition of well-being that would allow me to live life to the fullest, not just about having a toned body or running marathons.

A thorough assessment of my physical skills served as the foundation for determining my present level of fitness. I started off by testing my cardiovascular fitness by cycling, swimming, and running. I learned more about my stamina, heart rate, and endurance thanks to these exercises. I used weightlifting to gauge my strength and gradually increased the resistance to track my development. It was crucial to evaluate my flexibility and mobility because they frequently go unnoticed but are crucial to overall fitness. Dynamic stretching and yoga were now an essential part of my evaluation.

Monitoring my development in these areas was essential. I kept a workout notebook where I noted my successes, failures, and observations. This notebook acted as a resource for inspiration as well as a chronicle of my experience. It enabled me to set practical objectives and precisely gauge my progress.

I understood the need to examine my dietary practices and lifestyle choices in addition to physical examinations. After all, nutrition is crucial to overall fitness. I kept track of the macronutrient ratios, micronutrients, and water levels in my diet. This procedure identified areas for improvement, such as cutting back on processed foods, boosting the consumption of whole foods, and altering portion sizes. It was a game-changing move in the direction of a healthy diet.

In addition to nutrition, I evaluated my stress levels and sleep habits. I realized how important restful sleep and stress management were to healing and general well-being. I was able to address elements that might have been hindering my development thanks to this all-encompassing strategy.

There were times of doubt and frustration along this self-evaluation journey. There were always going to be obstacles, and progress was not always linear. But persistence and dedication to the process were crucial. I discovered how to enjoy minor successes, whether they involved going the extra mile, lifting more weight, or selecting a healthy dinner over fast food.

Measuring my level of fitness became a regular activity rather than a one-time project. I periodically went back to my assessments to monitor my development and revise my objectives. I was able to improve my workout regimen and modify it to better suit my changing requirements and goals thanks to this iterative process.

Setting Clear Goals

Any lifestyle adjustment can be difficult. Having a goal in mind gives many people something to strive for, inspires them to stay on course, and gives them a gauge of how well they are doing.

Setting realistic, well-thought-out goals will help you stay motivated and focused when trying to increase your physical activity.

Goal-setting for Physical Activity

You can use a few important ideas to guide how you set your physical activity objectives. These consist of:

Identify your long-term fitness goal

- Be reasonable: Your ultimate fitness goal can be to be in shape enough to compete on a specific date or to complete 10 laps of the pool. In any way, make this objective attainable. Keep in mind that the majority of us will never achieve supermodel or sportsman status. Consider what you are capable of. Goals should be written down.

- Be specific: Avoid making your final goal a blanket declaration like, "I want to lose weight." Create a metric for it. How many pounds do you aim to lose precisely?

- Pick a goal that matters and is significant to you alone, not to anyone else. For instance, you might find it challenging to stick with your fitness program over the long haul if your partner wants you to lose weight but you're content with how you look.

Learn how to reach your long-term fitness goal

Once you've chosen your fitness and health goal, you need to think about how you'll get there. Different approaches are needed for various fitness goals. For instance, in order to lose weight, you must routinely expend more calories than you ingest. An efficient plan might include:

- Opt for cardio exercises like walking.

- Work out for at least 30 minutes every day of the week, if not every day.

- Consume less junk food.

- Reduce food portions.

- Include more wholegrain foods, lean meats, fresh fruits and vegetables, low-fat dairy products, and fresh produce in your regular diet.

Set manageable, precise fitness targets

If you divide your main goal into smaller, more immediate mini-goals, you'll have a better chance of achieving it. Short-term goals are particular everyday habits or actions that point you in the direction of your long-term objective. Some suggestions are:

- Be aware of where you are starting from so that you may choose activities that are realistic and comfortable for you and progress gradually at a pace that feels suitable for you.

- Establish a fair deadline. For instance, if your goal is to lose 20kg, a realistic weight loss rate of 1kg of body fat every one to two weeks indicates you should give yourself 20 to 40 weeks to complete the task.

- Treat each of your workouts as a mini-goal. As an illustration, one micro goal might be to work out every day or most days of the week. Your motivation will increase as you complete more mini-goals.

Consult a professional if you are unclear about the best way to meet your unique fitness objectives. For instance, see your doctor, read through the fact sheets on the Better Health Channel, or talk to a personal trainer who is duly licensed, qualified, and certified in exercise physiology.

Regularly track your physical activity

Your mini-goals should be quantifiable. Make a plan for tracking your progress, and make sure to include every detail in a training journal.

- Track your development in tangible ways. Consider writing down the weight and repetitions for each exercise if you are weight training. Keep note of your weight loss if you are exercising to lose weight.

- Pick accurate metrics to gauge your advancement. For instance, bathroom scales don't differentiate between fat and muscle. It could be preferable to simply measure yourself with a tape measure or look at how your clothing fits.

- Use as many different methods as you can to keep track of your progress, and do so frequently—once a week, for example—by writing it down. For instance, if you exercise to lose weight, you might want to keep track of your workouts, daily dietary intake, and weekly measurements. Include unintended victories, such as having more energy or fitting into a smaller pair of trousers. Give yourself several opportunities to achieve.

- Honor your advancement.

Adapt your exercise to the environment as it changes

Your exercise regimen may be interrupted by life. Adapting to these changes entails:

- Consider strategies for handling disruptions. For instance, while on vacation you might not be able to exercise the way you usually do, but you can always go for a stroll or use the fitness center at the hotel.

- Keep working toward your fitness goals even if you are sick or injured. Instead, change the timeline for your ultimate goal. Create little goals to help you stay on track while you heal. For instance, even if you're too sick to exercise, you can still modify your diet. To stay motivated, note these mini-goals in your training journal.

- If reaching your fitness goal appears impossible, change your mini-goals and keep going.

Physical activity – Try not to be too hard on yourself

Your fitness goal could occasionally prove to be overly lofty. Consider the possibility that you are losing 0.5kg per week rather than 1 kg, and keep in mind that sometimes you may not drop any weight (muscular weighs more than fat). Instead, take a cognizance of how you feel. You are much more familiar with yourself than a set of scales.

- The most difficult months of a new workout regimen are generally the first few. Adjusting your short-term goals will help. Be persistent and have faith that things will get better.

- Honor all of your accomplishments, big or small. Even if your fitness goal is a little more challenging to achieve than you initially expected, making the commitment to a healthy lifestyle is an incredible accomplishment. Return to the beginning of your training journal to take in your progress.

- Have a backup fitness goal in mind. For instance, being able to jog for 20 minutes can be your secondary goal if your primary goal is to shed 20kg. This secondary objective being accomplished is still a huge triumph.

· Continue trying. You're worth the effort.

Designing Your Workout Routine

In all of its manifestations, fitness is a deeply individualized endeavor. We follow this approach to gradually accomplish our health and fitness goals. The development of a customized exercise regimen, a plan painstakingly made to match each of our specific requirements and goals, is essential to this trip. Let me walk you through my experience developing a training regimen, the lessons I've learned, and the impact a well-organized fitness plan can have.

My foray into fitness started with a trigger, a lightbulb moment that inspired me to travel this revolutionary path. It didn't happen all at once; rather, I gradually realized how crucial exercise and health were to my life. I knew the first step was to design a fitness regimen that would support my objectives as I thought about the changes I wanted to make.

My goals were well defined at the first stages of designing my training plan. I gave it some thought and asked myself what I wanted to accomplish. Was it a better overall state of health, muscle increase, weight loss, or enhanced endurance? I was able to establish definite, specific goals, which became the basis of my fitness journey.

One of the most important lessons I learned along this journey was that there is no one-size-fits-all training plan and that I must customize the routine to meet my needs. It's possible that what works for someone else won't work for me. I had to think about my degree of fitness, any existing medical concerns, and my preferences.

As I tried new workouts and activities, my training routine changed over time. I discovered that I liked a combination of cardio exercises like running and cycling, strength training with free weights and resistance bands, and the advantages of yoga for increasing flexibility. This variety kept my routine interesting and kept me from getting bored.

The importance of growth became clear to me as I carried on with my fitness adventure. My exercise program needed to change as my level of fitness increased; it could not stay the same. This means gradually stepping up the difficulty, length, or intensity of my workouts. Whether it was lifting bigger weights, covering longer distances on the run, or perfecting challenging yoga poses, I constantly documented my development.

One thing I learned was the value of rest and recovery in my exercise regimen. I understood that exerting too much effort without getting enough rest raised my risk of injury and led to burnout. To make sure my body had time to repair and regenerate, I incorporated rest days into my schedule and investigated recovery techniques like stretching, foam rolling, and meditation.

Consistency and discipline were the most important factors to consider when creating my workout plan. I discovered that dedication was necessary for success in fitness, as it is in any effort. There were times when motivation was low, but those were the times when discipline prevailed. I kept reminding myself of my objectives and the advancement I had achieved, which frequently renewed my motivation.

A Way of Life, Not a Fix

In the end, creating an exercise program helped me come to the startling insight that fitness is a lifetime commitment rather than a quick fix. It's not about getting somewhere, but about adopting a way of life that puts health and well-being first. My fitness regimen developed into a vital component of my daily life and a source of both mental and physical fortitude.

Monitoring Progress

Fitness and self-improvement journeys are intensely personal journeys filled with ups and downs, struggles, and victories. It's a route frequently followed with a certain goal in mind, whether it's getting in shape, losing excess weight, or just feeling better and more confident. Tracking progress, though, stands out as an essential tool in the complex tapestry of this trip. This frequently underrated tool has been the driving force behind my own fitness journey, providing direction, inspiration, and a real sense of accomplishment.

My entry into the world of fitness wasn't brought on by a single, paradigm-shifting insight. The need for and desire for a better lifestyle became apparent over time. I found that the first stage in my transformation was setting clear, defined goals amidst the cacophony of well-ness advice and fad diets. These goals served as the North Stars for my endeavors, giving them focus and direction.

But having specific goals wasn't enough. I wanted a way to track my development and a way to physically see how far I had come on this route. Thus, the idea of monitoring my success in my fitness quest was created.

Technology has made it possible to track development with a wide range of instruments. For me, my dependable buddy was a fitness app. I was able to log my workouts, keep track of my diet, and track changes in my body composition over time thanks to this digital ally. It turned my smartphone into a fitness command center and gave me access to a range of information that went beyond scale readings.

These measurements became my benchmarks. I rejoiced in every pound shed, every mile logged, and every percentage of weight lifted. I was able to see the minor successes that frequently go unnoticed by the human eye because of the measurement's profound potency. Even on days when the mirror didn't immediately confirm progress or when a workout felt especially challenging, the data revealed consistent advancement and small improvements.

However, tracking progress went beyond numbers. It explored the abstract facets of my journey. I kept a journal where I recorded my daily energy levels, how I felt after each workout, and how my clothes fit. These non-numerical indications provided a more complete view of my fitness journey, highlighting the fact that it was about more than just appearance.

Progress tracking was a collaborative effort that served as a regular reminder of responsibility and a strong incentive. It turned hazy fitness goals into concrete, quantifiable benchmarks. It forced me to keep the promises I had made to myself. The idea of maintaining or making progress served as an anchor, tethering me to my fitness regimen, when inspiration faltered and the pull of comfort tempted me to skip an exercise or indulge in bad habits.

Celebrating successes was maybe one of the most rewarding aspects of tracking progress. These successes were celebrated, whether it was a significant weight loss, running a longer distance, or setting a personal best in strength training. They encouraged me to keep pushing my boundaries by confirming the improvements I had made.

Chapter Four

Exercises and Specific Muscle Groups

The majority of us are aware of the benefits of regular exercise for our health, but we may not be sure where to begin or what activities are best. Exercise can take many various forms, and each one is beneficial to our health and quality of life in a different way. Training in aerobics, strength, and flexibility are the three main exercise modalities. They are all essential for maintaining health for as long as possible and each has unique advantages.

We frequently forget to include strength training in our fitness regimens. Contrary to popular belief, strength training isn't only for guys, it's not just for young people, and it's not just for when you're trying to bulk up your muscles. At any age, strength training is beneficial for everyone, and getting started is simpler than you might think. This chapter will explain the importance and advantages of strength training, provide you with a general outline of exercises, and inspire you with suggestions for how to include it in your daily routine.

Upper Body

The human body is a complex work of engineering, with every component having a specific function. The upper body occupies a specific place of significance in the world of fitness. It is in the physical realm where functionality, grace, and strength come together. The importance of the upper body, its amazing complexity, and its transforming ability are discussed below.

The Upper Body: A Complex Marvel

The interesting variety of muscles, joints, and bones that make up the upper body are intimately interwoven to allow for a large range of mobility and functionality. It is the driving force behind crucial daily tasks like lifting groceries, using a keyboard and reaching up to get items from high shelves. It also has a crucial impact on how athletes perform, whether it is the grace of a ballet dancer, the strength of a weightlifter, or the delicacy of a tennis player.

The upper body is made up mostly of many important parts:

Shoulders: The collarbone (clavicle), shoulder blade (scapula), and upper arm bone (humerus) make up the complicated shoulder girdle. It gives the upper body mobility and stability, enabling motions like lifting, pushing, and reaching.

Arms: The workhorses of the upper body are the arms, which house important muscular groups like the biceps and triceps. They make it easier to lift, transport, and manipulate objects—essential tasks.

Chest: Pectoral muscles in the chest are necessary for hugs and pushing motions. In addition to being practical, well-developed chest muscles also help to create an attractive upper body.

Back: The muscles of the back, particularly the latissimus dorsi and trapezius, give stability and power to a variety of upper body movements. They are important for tugging and lifting tasks.

Neck: Although frequently disregarded, the muscles in the neck support the head and are crucial for upholding appropriate posture. They contribute to both practical and aesthetically pleasing movements.

Strength and Usefulness

The upper body's ability to produce strength and functionality is one of its main purposes. The muscles in the upper body are used for a wide variety of activities, from everyday chores like combing your hair to more difficult ones like doing pull-ups or using an instrument.

There are more benefits to upper body strength than just looking good or being able to lift a lot of weight. It has a direct impact on life quality. Strong upper body muscles assist in preventing injuries, promote functionality overall, and improve posture. In order to keep our independence as we age and carry out necessary chores without trouble, a strong upper body is necessary.

Visual Appeal and Self-Assurance

The upper body plays a significant part in defining our body's beauty in addition to its utilitarian elements. An attractive figure has sculpted shoulders, defined arms, and a well-developed chest. This aesthetic quality inspires confidence and self-assurance in many people. Having a positive body image and feeling physically fit can increase self-esteem.

The Upper Body in Athletics and Sports

The upper body is frequently the focus in the realm of sports and athletics. It is the driving force behind shot put throws, what propels a sprinter's arm motion, and what enables a gymnast to perform graceful routines on the uneven bars. The cornerstone of athletic performance, the upper body's strength, endurance, and agility are essential for succeeding in a variety of sports.

Training and Development

Training and growth are crucial to maximizing the upper body's capabilities. Exercises that target the shoulders, arms, chest, back, and neck are part of a well-rounded upper-body workout routine. These exercises can include weightlifting movements like bench presses and rows as well as body-weight workouts like pushups and pullups. Yoga, Pilates, and functional training regimens can also improve flexibility and mobility.

To avoid injuries and maximize gains, it's critical to approach upper body training with the right form and technique. The secret to continuous improvement is a progressive strategy that steadily increases weight and intensity.

Lower Body

The lower body is the foundation of the human body's symphony. The hips, thighs, knees, and calves of the lower body are more than just a structural support system. It serves as the foundation for many of our daily tasks and sports endeavors. It is a force house of strength, agility, and movement. Let's look into the significance of the lower body, its amazing intricacy, and its crucial function in maintaining our physical health.

The Surprising Complexity of the Lower Body

The lower body is a biomechanical and engineering marvel. A vast variety of movements and activities are made possible by the body's complex network of muscles, bones, and joints. The lower body acts as the focal point of our physical talents, controlling everything from the straightforward motion of walking to the explosive movements of running, jumping, and dancing.

Hips and Thighs: Femur (the thigh bone) and pelvis are connected by the hip joint, one of the biggest and strongest in the body. It permits a great range of motion, making it possible to perform motions like walking, running, squatting, and lunging. These motions are made possible by the muscles of the hips and thighs, specifically the quadriceps, hamstrings, and glutes, which are also crucial for supporting the body's weight-bearing activities.

Knees: The knee joints serve as pivotal hinges and are located between the thigh bone and the shinbone. They make movements like walking, climbing stairs, and cycling possible by enabling the lower leg's flexion and extension. The coordination of ligaments and muscles, including the quadriceps and hamstrings, is essential for maintaining the stability of the knee.

Calves: The gastrocnemius and soleus muscles in the calves are in charge of the ankle's plantarflexion, which enables us to propel ourselves off the ground when walking or running. Balance and stability also heavily rely on strong calves.

Power and Flexibility

The lower body is a strength-producing machine. In addition to helping it move, its muscles also help it stay balanced and stable. Activities requiring bending, lifting, or carrying heavy loads require strong quadriceps, hamstrings, and glutes. We can complete these duties with ease and without danger of injury.

Another characteristic of the lower body is mobility. Particularly the hip joint provides a tremendous range of mobility, enabling us to pivot, twist, and move in different directions. For athletic performance, practical movements, and general flexibility, adequate hip mobility is crucial.

Sports and Athletic Capability

The foundation of athletic ability is the lower body. Sports like running, jumping, cycling, and soccer are propelled by it. Whether a sprinter explodes out of the starting blocks or a basketball player leaps for a dunk, strong, explosive lower-body muscles are essential for producing power and speed.

All types of athletes are aware of the value of lower body conditioning. To improve their lower body strength and explosiveness, they devote time to workouts like squats, deadlifts, and plyometrics.

Training and Development

Training and growth are crucial if you want to use the lower body to its maximum capacity. Exercises that target various muscle groups are included in lower body training. Some of the fundamental exercises for developing lower body strength include squats, lunges, leg presses, and deadlifts. Additionally, exercises like yoga and stretching programs help improve the flexibility and mobility of the lower body.

In order to avoid injuries and maintain efficient muscle engagement, proper form and technique are essential when working the lower body. To see persistent improvement, choose a progressive strategy that gradually raises the weight and intensity.

Core Strength

When someone is trying to get in shape, the attention is frequently drawn to their biceps, chest, and legs. However, a silent hero, the core, is concealed beneath these visible signs of strength. It is the hidden source of strength and vigor, the foundation upon which all motions and endeavors rely.

I was dreaming of having a lean, strong figure, like many others. My early workouts focused on developing observable muscles, frequently ignoring the core. After all, the core was still hidden beneath many layers of abdominal fat, seemingly unimportant to the appearance I was going for.

However, after suffering a lower back injury, my viewpoint on core strength changed. The discomfort served as a wake-up call, a clear reminder that the core is important for functional strength and overall well-being in addition to providing washboard abs.

The core, I learned, reaches deep into the torso and includes the muscles in the lower back, hips, and pelvis in addition to the abdominal muscles. It serves as the body's stabilizing center, similar to the base of a strong structure. Everyday actions like bending, lifting, twisting, and even sitting become difficult and risk damage without a strong and solid core.

I became aware of core training's transforming effect as I dove further into it. A solid core is essential for improving athletic performance as well as injury prevention. It serves as the building block for power and strength in a variety of exercises, including lifting heavy objects, long-distance running, and dynamic yoga positions. It is the foundation of stability and balance, enabling us to retain balance when engaging in a variety of tasks including standing on one leg, negotiating rough terrain, or conquering challenging dance routines.

My core exercises progressed from straightforward crunches to a comprehensive strategy that focused on all the muscles in this crucial region. Russian twists, bird dogs, planks, and bridges all became a part of my routine. These workouts worked the deeper muscles, such as the transverse abdominis and multifidus, which are crucial for spinal stability in addition to the visible rectus abdominis.

As I improved in my core training, I noticed real advantages outside of the gym. I felt more grounded and secure during daily activities, and my posture improved. I started to feel less vulnerable and uncomfortable because of my lower back issue. Whether I was carrying heavy items or taking part in outdoor activities, I could move with assurance.

My athletic ability also improved significantly. During workouts, I had more strength and stamina, and my balance and coordination also got better. My core strength was a game-changer whether I was hiking up rocky trails or taking part in a friendly game of soccer.

Total-Body Exercises

The holistic approach to fitness is best exemplified by total body exercises. These exercises work for many muscle groups concurrently, in contrast to programs that isolate particular muscle groups. The goal is to develop total strength, endurance, flexibility, and balance, laying the groundwork for a physique with a variety of muscle groups.

Why Whole-Body Workouts Are Important

Total-body exercises have a number of advantages that improve general health and fitness, including:

Efficiency: They make the most of your workout time by focusing on several muscle groups at once. You spend less time working out while still getting a thorough exercise.

Functional Strength: Exercises for the entire body foster functional strength, which leads to better performance in daily tasks. Being able to lift, carry, and move objects effectively and securely is a sign of functional strength.

Prevention of Muscle Imbalances: These workouts lessen the possibility of developing muscle imbalances, which can result in injuries or discomfort.

Variety: Total body exercises use a variety of activities, minimizing monotony and maintaining training interest. The body must continually adapt to and advance in response to this variation.

Cardiovascular Benefits: A lot of complete body exercises have cardiovascular components that serve to strengthen the heart, increase endurance, and promote fat loss.

Improved Flexibility and Balance: Yoga or stretching exercises, which are frequently incorporated into total-body workouts, improve flexibility and balance. This improves general mobility and helps to prevent injuries.

Stronger Mind-Body Connection: Total body workouts frequently place an emphasis on mindfulness and mental attention.

The Complete Approach to Total Body Exercises

Let's now examine the best ways to perform total-body exercises:

Step 1: Warm-Up (5-10 minutes)

Start by lightly warming up your muscles and joints. The best exercises include dynamic stretching, jumping jacks, and stationary jogging.

Step 2: Sample Exercises

Here are a few examples of exercises to incorporate into your total-body training program:

1. **Squats:**

    - Place your feet shoulder-width apart as you stand.

    - Squat down by bringing your hips back and bending your knees.

    - Keep your back straight and your chest up.

    - Straightening your legs will bring you back to the starting position.

    - Shoot for three sets of 10 to 12 reps.

2. **Push-Ups:**

    - Place your hands shoulder-width apart in a plank stance to begin.

    - Squat down until your chest is nearly parallel to the floor.

    - Raise yourself back up to where you were.

    - Strive for 3 sets of 8 – 10 repetitions.

3.   **Lunges:**

- Step out with your feet hip-width apart.

- Take a forward step with one leg, then squat down until your knees are at a 90-degree angle.

- Return to the starting position by pushing up, then repeat with the opposite leg.

- For each leg, aim for 3 sets of 10 – 12 reps.

4.   **Plank:**

- Start with your arms extended in the push-up position.

- Engage your core and keep your body in a straight line from head to heels.

- Remain in this position for 30 to 60 seconds.

- Try to get 3 sets.

5.   **Deadlifts (with barbells or dumbbells)**

- Hold weights in front of your thighs while standing with your feet hip-width apart.

- Maintain a straight back while bending at the hips and knees to reduce the weight.

- Resuming your upright stance.

- Strive for 3 sets of 8 – 10 repetitions.

Step 3: Cool Off (5 – 10 Minutes)

You should chill down after your full-body workout. Target the main muscle areas you worked on during your workout with static stretching movements.

Step 4: Recuperation and Rest

Between total-body workouts, give your body some time to heal. In general, 48 hours of rest is advised to provide muscles enough time to recover and strengthen.

Chapter Five

Utilizing Strength Training to Increase Fat Burn

High-intensity Interval Training (HIIT) has become increasingly popular in the fitness industry, changing how we perceive exercise and pushing the limits of what our bodies are capable of. Fundamentals of HIIT were key components to my own road to a better, more energetic life.

The HIIT Revolution: A Fitness Paradigm Shift

A workout routine known as HIIT is characterized by quick bursts of all-out, intense exertion followed by brief intervals of rest or active recovery. This ostensibly straightforward idea has changed the exercise landscape by providing a workout that is not only effective but also incredibly efficient. The idea that lengthier, moderate-intensity workouts are the only way to get healthy is challenged by HIIT. Shorter, more intense workouts have been demonstrated to produce outstanding outcomes in terms of cardiovascular health, fat loss, and general strength.

Shifting From Been Doubtful to a Believer

My initial exposure to HIIT was accompanied by doubt. Like many others, I had been trained to think that lengthier, steady-state cardio sessions were the ideal for getting in shape. It seems contradictory to shorten my workout while boosting its intensity. I decided to attempt HIIT out of curiosity, and that choice would permanently alter the way I saw fitness.

The first HIIT workout was absolutely revelatory. The intensity was thrilling and exhausting at the same time, driving me to the edge of my stamina. I had finished a workout that left me out of breath, bathed in perspiration, and with a great sense of success in just 20 minutes. It was very different from the drawn-out, boring aerobic workouts to which I had grown accustomed.

I started to experience the transformational impact of HIIT as I continued to incorporate it into my training routine. The results I got were overwhelming. Not only did my cardiovascular fitness significantly improve, but I also saw a considerable drop in body fat. I felt stronger and more agile during daily chores as my muscular tone improved.

The Science of HIIT's Effectiveness

The effectiveness of HIIT is validated by scientific studies and is not only anecdotal. When the body is in an oxygen-depleted state from high-intensity intervals, it must work harder to recover during rest times. Too much post-exercise oxygen consumption, as it is been called results to a rapid rate of burning calories which take place when the activity is ongoing. In short, HIIT provides a powerful mix of benefits for cardiovascular conditioning and fat-burning in a shorter amount of time.

HIIT: A Flexible Exercise Program

The adaptability of HIIT is one of its amazing qualities. It can be modified to accommodate different fitness levels and objectives. HIIT may be customized to meet your needs, whether you're an experienced athlete looking to improve performance or a novice ready to begin a fitness journey. Jumping jacks, burpees, and other conventional exercises can be used, as well as more advanced routines involving tools like kettlebells and battle ropes.

Metabolic Resistance Training

There are many different training approaches as a result of the search for efficient and effective workouts. Among them, Metabolic Resistance Training (MRT) has distinguished itself as a force to be reckoned with. It provides a dynamic approach that not only tests the body but also speeds up metabolic processes for the best fat loss and muscle building.

Metabolic Resistance Training's Fundamentals

An organized, high-intensity training method called metabolic resistance training mixes strength training with cardiovascular activities. The main objective of MRT is to stimulate numerous muscle groups while maintaining an elevated heart rate, producing a dual effect that increases strength and burns calories. MRT adopts a holistic approach, encouraging total-body involvement for a thorough fitness transformation as opposed to conventional workouts that concentrate on single muscle groups.

The Metabolic Boost in the Science of MRT

The potential of metabolic resistance training to speed up the body's metabolism is what makes it effective. Too much post-exercise oxygen consumption, or which is also known as EPOC, is an afterburn effect caused by MRT's high intensity, and meanwhile this raises heart rate and increases what oxygen requires. This implies that even after a workout, the body continues to burn calories as it tries to go back to how it was before the activity. The ability of MRT to burn fat is significantly influenced by this metabolic increase.

The Positive Effect on Fitness

MRT attracts exercise enthusiasts of all levels with a variety of transforming advantages:

1. Efficiency: MRT mixes cardio and strength training, allowing for a more thorough exercise in less time.

2. Fat reduction: The increased heart rate during MRT encourages the burning of fat reserves for energy, which helps to improve efficient fat reduction.

3. Muscle Gain: MRT promotes the growth and toning of muscles by using resistance workouts to work a variety of muscle groups.

4. Metabolic Boost: The EPOC afterburn effect helps with weight management by continuing to burn calories after the workout.

5. Functional Strength: MRT puts an emphasis on compound movements that increase functional strength, making daily tasks simpler and more effective.

6. Variety: MRT provides countless exercise variants that break up the monotony of a workout and promote the growth of lean muscle.

7. Cardiovascular Health: The MRT's cardiovascular component improves stamina and heart health.

The Organization of an MRT Workout

A typical MRT workout has the following format:

Circuit Training: MRT frequently uses circuit-style workouts, in which a number of exercises are carried out one after the other with little break in between.

High Intensity: Each workout is performed vigorously, putting the heart and muscles to the test.

Resistance Exercises: To work out the primary muscle groups, resistance exercises including squats, lunges, push-ups, and rows are frequently used.

Cardio Intervals: To keep the heart rate raised, cardiovascular activities like jumping jacks, mountain climbers, and sprints are inserted between sets of resistance training.

Short Rest Times: To keep the heart rate constant and maximize the metabolic effect, rest times are kept brief.

Strength Training vs. Cardio for Fat Loss

In the field of fitness, pursuing fat loss is a frequent objective. However, the method for reaching this objective frequently causes controversy: Strength training or cardio? The dynamics of cardio and strength training, their individual effects on fat reduction, and the significance of striking the correct balance between the two will then be discussed. We'll also go over a few examples of each form of training to highlight the benefits and contrasts between them.

Sweating Out – The Cardiovascular Equation

Cardiovascular exercise, or cardio, refers to a group of exercises that increase heart rate and maintain it for an extended length of time. These are examples of cardio exercises: Running, cycling, swimming, and aerobics. Due to their capacity to produce a caloric deficit, cardio exercises are typically linked to calorie burning and fat loss.

Sample Cardio Workout: Running

- Activity: Running either outside or on a treadmill.

- Duration: 30 to 60 minutes.

- Intensity: Moderate to high, moving at a steady pace.

- Caloric Burn: Running can burn between 300 – 600 calories per hour, depending on factors including speed and body weight.

Strength Training – Building the Fat-Burning Engine

On the other hand, resistance exercises that target particular muscle groups are part of strength training. Weightlifting, bodyweight exercises, and resistance band workouts are some of these exercises. Although it may not burn as many calories during the session as cardio, strength training is essential for gaining lean muscle growth.

Sample Strength Training Workout: Bodyweight Exercises

- Activity: Planks, lunges, squats, and push-ups using only your body weight.

- Duration: 20 to 30 minutes.

- Intensity: Moderate to high, emphasizing correct form and deliberate motion.

The Fat Loss Dilemma – Cardio vs. Strength Training

The differences in their unique systems are often the crux of the argument between cardio and strength training for fat loss:

1. Caloric Burn: Cardio increases calorie expenditure when exercising, helping to create the caloric deficit required for fat loss.

2. Muscle Building: Strength training helps to develop lean muscle, which raises the resting metabolic rate. As a result, even while you're at rest, you burn more calories.

3. Afterburn Effect: Excess Post-Exercise Oxygen Consumption (EPOC), a side effect of strength training, causes the body to continue burning calories after a workout.

Finding the Balance – The Synergy of Cardio and Strength Training

It's important to realize that cardio and strength training can work in tandem to effectively burn fat rather than seeing them as opposing forces. The best outcomes can be achieved with a well-rounded strategy that includes both kinds of training. This is how:

1. Days Dedicated to Cardio: On these days, concentrate on cardio exercises to reduce your caloric intake.

2.   Strength-Training Days: Include strength training to increase metabolism and develop lean muscular mass.

3.   High-Intensity Interval Training (HIIT): HIIT is a powerful fat-loss technique because it incorporates components of both cardio and strength training.

4.   Nutrition: To accelerate fat reduction, combine your workouts with a healthy, calorie-restricted diet.

Advanced Methods and Tips

Fitness excellence is a journey that changes over time. It's a journey distinguished by ongoing learning and development, where sophisticated strategies and tactics serve as stepping stones for achieving new heights.

Progressive Overload

The idea of gradual overload is at the core of advanced training. According to this idea, you must gradually put more demands on your body in order to show improvement over time. Mind you, this can be carried out in diverse of ways:

Increasing resistance: Gradually upping the resistance level pushes your muscles and encourages growth whether you're using weights, your body weight, or resistance bands.

Changing the reps and sets: Changing up your workout routine's repetition and set counts can promote strength and muscle growth. Drop sets, supersets, and pyramid exercises are advanced techniques that increase intensity and variation.

Periodization: This is the division of your training into cycles, each with a distinct goal. With this method, progress is continual and plateaus are avoided.

Tempo variations: You can improve muscle engagement and promote growth by changing the tempo of your lifts, such as by slowing down the eccentric (falling) component of a movement.

Pushing Boundaries: Advanced Exercises

Exercises that are more difficult and sophisticated are frequently incorporated into routines for advanced training. These exercises demand remarkable stability and coordination while working a variety of muscle groups and enhancing functional strength. Examples comprise:

Olympic Lifts: Exercises like the clean and jerk and snatch need extraordinary mobility, precision, and explosive force.

Calisthenics: Advanced bodyweight workouts that challenge your strength-to-weight ratio and core stability include muscle-ups, handstand push-ups, and front levers.

Plyometrics: Activities like box jumps and depth jumps improve agility and explosive force.

Complexes with kettlebells: The kettlebell swings, snatches, and Turkish get-ups put your strength, stamina, and coordination to the test.

Advanced Tips – Fine-Tuning Your Approach

Advanced fitness lovers rely on sophisticated tactics to maximize their training in addition to workouts and resistance levels:

Periodization of nutrition: Align your calorie intake and macronutrient ratios with your training cycles to support your objectives.

Active recovery: To improve post-workout recovery and lower the chance of injury, use active recovery techniques like foam rolling, yoga, and mobility exercises.

Mind-body relationship: Create a strong mental-muscular link to ensure that each repetition is carried out precisely and purposefully, optimizing muscle activation.

Rest and sleep: Give your body enough time to heal and grow between tough workouts by prioritizing good sleep.

Mental resilience: Develop mental toughness, discipline, and focus to get through difficult workouts and remain dedicated to your goals.

Personalization – Your Individual Journey

Although sophisticated methods and advice are effective tools, it's critical to keep in mind that achieving fitness is a highly individualized process. Remember that solution that worked for one person might not be suitable for another. It's imperative to adjust your strategy to fit your particular goals, body type, and interests.

Chapter Six

Injury Prevention and Recovery

Be aware that the importance of perseverance, commitment, and pushing oneself to the limit is unwavering in the field of fitness. We frequently hear the sayings "no pain, no gain" and "keep grinding." While these maxims undoubtedly have their place, rest and recovery are another crucial component of fitness that are just as important, if not more so. The fundamental value of rest and recuperation in a fitness journey is explored below, along with how my own experience highlights the significance of these frequently disregarded components.

It's simple to get sucked into the never-ending grind of training when trying to achieve our fitness objectives, whether they be gaining strength, increasing endurance, or losing excess weight. I was previously caught up in this mindset as well. When I first started working out, I had an unquenchable desire to get better and pushed myself constantly. I thought that the more training I did, the quicker my goals would be attained.

But eventually, this unyielding strategy brought about results I hadn't expected. My body started to complain. My exercise regimen began to be plagued by persistent exhaustion, bothersome injuries, and a lasting feeling of burnout. It served as a wake-up call and a sharp reminder that I had failed to prioritize rest and recovery, two essential components of fitness.

Rest and recovery are essential components of a successful fitness journey, not evidence of weakness. Here's why they're important:

Muscle Repair and Growth: When you exercise hard, your muscles are stressed and microscopic damage occurs. These muscles rebuild and strengthen themselves during the interval of rest and recuperation. Without enough sleep, the body cannot efficiently repair itself, which causes progress to stall.

Injury Prevention: In the field of fitness, overtraining is a major cause of injuries. Overuse injuries are less likely when people get enough rest so that their bodies can recuperate from the physical strain of activity.

Hormonal Balance: Prolonged and strenuous exercise can mess with your hormones, which can cause problems including cortisol imbalances and sleep problems. A good night's sleep helps hormone balance return.

Mental Rejuvenation: Being fit requires more than just physical strength; it also requires mental toughness. Rest and recuperation give the mind the room it needs to keep one's excitement and drive for long-term objectives.

Performance Boosting: Athletes at the highest levels of competition prioritize recovery as a way to improve their performance, contrary to the notion that more training results in better performance. The body can perform at its best during workouts and contests when it has a good night's sleep.

This has taught me the value of striking a balance between exertion and recovery. I came to the conclusion that the quality of the workouts, not the quantity, is what makes a difference. My growth was accelerated by including rest days and giving my body time to recover. I found that after a break from training, I was stronger, more concentrated, and more determined than before.

I give this counsel to individuals starting their fitness adventures or who are already far along the way: emphasize rest and recuperation as ardently as you do your workouts. Pay attention to your body, spot overtraining symptoms, and welcome rest days not as setbacks but as necessary advancements. Whether it's active rehabilitation, yoga, stretching, or simply taking a day off, find a balance that works for you.

Stretching and Flexibility

i. **The Usefulness of Flexibility and Stretching**

- Increased Range of Motion: Flexibility allows joints and muscles to move more freely, which improves functional mobility.

- Injury Prevention: Muscles and tendons that are in good condition are less likely to be strained or torn during physical activity.

- Lessened Muscular Tension: Stretching helps reduce muscular tension and discomfort, which promotes general relaxation.

- Better Posture: Flexibility helps maintain good posture, which lowers the risk of musculoskeletal problems.

- Balance and Coordination: Stretching enhances balance and coordination, which are essential for daily activities and athletic performance.

- Stress Reduction: By releasing endorphins, stretching promotes relaxation and stress reduction.

ii.   **The Science of Stretching**

Targeting particular muscles or muscle groups while maintaining a stretch in a static position is known as static stretching.

- Dynamic Stretching: This technique involves adding movement to stretches to increase flexibility and warm up muscles.

- Proprioceptive Neuromuscular Facilitation (PNF): A more sophisticated method for increasing flexibility that involves stretching, contracting, and relaxing different muscle groups.

- Ballistic Stretching: This type of stretching involves bouncing or jerking motions and is not advised owing to the possibility of harm.

iii.   **Useful Methods for Increasing Flexibility**

Shoulders and Neck

Neck Tilt: Gently tilt your head from side to side while holding each stretch for 15 to 30 seconds.

Shoulder Stretch: To extend your shoulders and chest, clasp your hands behind your back and slowly elevate your arms.

Upper Body:

Triceps Stretch: Raise one arm overhead, bend at the elbow, and extend the opposing hand behind your head.

Chest Opener: Interlace your fingers behind your back as you slowly lift your arms upward.

Lower Body:

Hamstring Stretch: To stretch your hamstrings, sit on the ground with one leg outstretched and toes pointing upward. For 15 to 30 seconds, reach for your toes and hold.

Quad Stretch: Stand on one leg and gradually bring the other heel toward your buttocks.

Back and Core:

Cat-Cow Stretch: Arc your back upward (like a cat) and then downward (like a cow) while on your hands and knees.

Child's Pose: Stretch your back and shoulders by sitting back on your heels with your arms out in front of you.

Hips and Glutes:

Pigeon Pose: Start in a plank position, then bring one knee forward, bending it such that the outside of the shin is on the floor.

Calves and Ankles:

Calf Stretch: Stand with one foot in front of the other while maintaining a straight back leg.

iv.　**Making Stretching a Part of Your Routine**

- Pre-workout: Warm up your muscles and get them ready for exercise by performing dynamic stretches.

- Post-workout: Concentrate on static stretching to increase flexibility and relieve tension in the muscles.

- Yoga and Pilates: These are fantastic complements to your regimen since they place an emphasis on flexibility and balance.

- Regularity: It's important to be consistent. Give stretching and flexibility exercises some of your daily or at least weekly time.

v.   **A Stretching Plan for Particular Activities**

- Running: When running, concentrate on leg stretches to lengthen your stride and lower your chance of injury.

- Weightlifting: To speed recovery, focus on the muscle regions that were worked throughout your weightlifting routine.

- Sedentary Work: To counteract the negative effects of extended sitting, stretch frequently to avoid postural problems.

The Techniques of Preventing Injuries

Do you know that the pursuit of strength, endurance, and general wellness in the context of fitness and physical activity is frequently accompanied by the inherent risk of injuries? However, these hazards can be considerably reduced with a comprehensive set of injury avoidance techniques.

i.   **Knowledge of Injury Causes**

One can only propose solutions to problems that are already known, so it is important to understand the primary causes of fitness-related injuries before diving into prevention strategies:

- Overuse: Repeated stress on muscles and joints as a result of excessive or ineffective training methods.

- Muscular Imbalances: Injuries can result from muscle imbalances, which occur when some muscle groups are noticeably stronger or weaker than their antagonistic counterparts.

- Poor Technique: Muscles and joints can become strained when workouts are performed incorrectly or with poor form.

- Poor Warm-Up and Cool-Down Techniques: Injury risk can be increased by improperly warming up and cooling down the body before exercise.

- Insufficient Rest and Recovery: Overuse injuries can result from not giving the body enough time to repair and rejuvenate.

ii.   **Injury Prevention Techniques: Steps You Can Take To Protect Your Fitness Journey**

1. *Suitable Warm-Up and Cool-Down*

   o Warm-Up: Perform gentle aerobics for 5 to 10 minutes to improve blood flow and prime muscles for workouts.

   o Dynamic Stretches: To improve mobility, incorporate dynamic stretches like arm circles, hip rotations, and leg swings.

o Cool Down: After your workout, stretch your muscles in a static position to increase flexibility and relieve tension.

2. *Technique and Form*

- o Education: Gain knowledge about good exercise methods from reliable sources, trainers, or fitness classes.

- o Progression: Gradually up the intensity of your workouts to let your body get used to the new motions.

- o Focus: During workouts, pay special attention to your form, stressing controlled movements.

3. *Strength and Balance Training*

- o Full-Body Workouts: Incorporate exercises that target all major muscle groups to maintain balance.

- o Core Stability: Strengthen your core to promote good posture and lower your chance of back issues.

4. *Flexibility and Mobility*

- o Consistently Stretching: Regularly stretch your muscles to increase flexibility and prevent muscle imbalances.

- o Yoga and Mobility Exercises: These two exercises can increase your general flexibility.

5. *Rest and Recovery*

- o Rest Days: Include rest days in your schedule to give your body time to repair and recover.

- o Sleep: Make this a top priority because it is crucial for muscle restoration and general recuperation.

6. *Pay Attention to Your Body*

- o Recognize pain: Know the difference between normal muscular aches and pain that could be an injury.

- o Rest When Necessary: Take Time to relax when it's necessary: If you're in pain or uncomfortable, take time to relax and, if necessary, get medical help.

7. *Nutrition and Hydration*

- o Balanced Diet: Give your body the nutrition it needs by consuming a balanced diet to enhance muscle and tissue regeneration.

- o Hydration: Keep your body well hydrated to keep your muscles functioning and avoid cramps.

8. *Gradual Progression*

- o Incremental Increases: To avoid overuse injuries, gradually increase the intensity, duration, or weight of your workouts.

9. *Regular Check-Ins*

o Physical Assessments: Examine your physical state on a regular basis to spot any new problems or imbalances.

o Professional Guidance: For examinations and individualized injury prevention techniques, seek the advice of a physical therapist or trainer.

10. *The Right Footwear and Equipment*

o Proper Shoes: Make an investment in supportive, high-quality athletic shoes that are appropriate for your particular activity.

o Protective Equipment: For activities where there is a higher risk of harm, wear protective equipment, such as helmets or joint supports.

iii. **Matching Your Prevention to Your Fitness Objectives**

- Cardiovascular Exercises: Pay close attention to dynamic warm-ups, escalating intensity gradually, and appropriate footwear.

- Strength training: Be sure to maintain proper form and balance, gradually increase the weights, and get enough recovery.

- Sports and Agility Training: Include sports-specific exercises and drills while putting an emphasis on agility and balance.

iv.   **Post-Injury Recovery**

- Seek Professional Assistance: If hurt, speak with a doctor or physical therapist to receive an accurate diagnosis and a treatment plan.

- Follow Medical Advice: To guarantee a full recovery, follow the advised treatment and rehabilitation programs.

Chapter Seven

Building a Sustainable Lifestyle

Juggling a variety of activities is frequently required in the quest for physical fitness and a balanced, healthy lifestyle. Strength training is one of them and is the foundation of physical health. Finding the right balance between strength training and other activities, however, may be a difficult but extremely gratifying task.

The appeal of strength training, for many fitness aficionados, including myself, is found in its capacity for transformation. It is certainly alluring to be able to develop lean muscle, functional strength, and overall physical toughness. It's simple to get caught up in a single fitness activity while pursuing these advantages, neglecting other pursuits that add to a balanced life.

This fine balance is embodied in my own life's path. The promise of toned muscles and enhanced power first drew me into the world of strength training as well. It was intoxicating to achieve personal bests and observe how my body changed. You can imagine that as time went on, I started to realize that my life was becoming disconnected from other areas due to my single-minded attention.

The realization that I had been skipping out on activities that used to bring me so much delight served as a wake-up call. Even the simple joy of a leisurely bike ride had become uncommon, as had hiking in the vast outdoors, playing recreational sports with friends, and other similar activities. The advantages of these activities for my mental and emotional health had been relegated to the background, and my social life had suffered.

This insight caused me to reconsider how I approach fitness. I started to realize that strength training should enhance my life rather than take over. Finding harmony between them was more important than picking one path over another.

What I learned about juggling strength training with other hobbies is as follows:

1.   Variety in Physical Demands: Participating in a range of activities puts diverse muscle groups and movement patterns to the test, lowering the likelihood of overuse injuries and enhancing general functional fitness.

2.   Mental and Emotional Well-being: Diverse hobbies provide your mind and heart a break from the strain of rigorous muscular training. The delight of learning new skills or simply taking in the outdoors can be a potent antidote to the stress of intense exercise.

3.   Social Connection: Engaging in team sports or group activities strengthens social links and builds a feeling of community, which may be gratifying and inspiring.

4.   Longevity: Variety in your physical activities encourages sustained involvement in fitness. Because each activity has a different set of difficulties and benefits, it lowers the likelihood of burnout.

5.   Goal Flexibility: By balancing various activities, fitness goals can be formed and modified with flexibility. You can adjust to shifting conditions and tastes thanks to it.

I rediscovered the excitement of trekking through pristine forests, the thrill of a friendly tennis match, and the simple pleasure of cycling along gorgeous roads on my own journey of juggling strength training with other interests. These pursuits not only improved my life but also restored the equilibrium of my mind and emotions that I had been lacking.

Intentionality and adaptation are essential for striking this equilibrium. It involves understanding the importance of each activity in enhancing your overall well-being and designing a fitness regimen that enables them to coexist peacefully. It's also important to realize that your path to fitness is dynamic and ever-evolving, and it may include a wide range of activities.

Keeping Up Your Results

A fantastic accomplishment that requires commitment, persistence, and hard effort is reaching fitness objectives. However, the struggle to retain the outcomes that have been worked so hard for is frequently overlooked.

Once upon a time, after gaining amazing improvements, including a slimmer physique, increased strength, and newfound confidence, via persistent effort and unrelenting devotion, the question that set in was "How could I maintain these results over the long run as I basked in the fulfillment of my accomplishments?"

A change in viewpoint is necessary to maintain fitness outcomes. It's important to embrace the journey as a continuous process rather than resting on one's laurels. I came to the conclusion that my way of thinking needed to change as I moved toward my goals. I changed my focus from being wholly on the results to being wholly on the process. I was aware that the path was ongoing and that I needed to maintain my dedication. The regularity that fuelled my advancement remained the foundation of upkeep. Regular exercise, mindful eating, and self-care practices became essential components of my regimen.

Our bodies and lives modify themselves just like the seasons. I understood that my exercise regimen needed to change to reflect these changes. I welcomed variation in my workouts, tried out new things to do, and modified my dietary strategy accordingly. I realized that my objectives should change as my aspirations do. I established new goals that were consistent with my ongoing path once specific milestones were attained.

I came to see that fitness couldn't exist independently; it needed to fit into my lifestyle. Whether it was walking, stretching, or engaging in active hobbies, I made decisions to incorporate exercise into my everyday life. Nutrition, mind you, was crucial to both obtaining and maintaining results. I concentrated on healthy, sustainable eating habits that fed my body without depriving it.

I also understood that working too hard without enough rest could result in burnout. To ensure my body's adaptability, I gave sleep, stress reduction, and active recovery techniques top priority.

The voyage will have peaks and down points. I looked at them as chances for improvement rather than as a source of discouragement. I discovered self-compassion and the value of the journey's ups and downs.

My experience with holding onto results is proof of the significant changes that may take place when we embrace the continual nature of fitness. Instead of focusing on getting somewhere, we should strive to live a life in which being healthy is an essential aspect of who we are.

It takes a combination of commitment and adaptation to maintain results. Knowing that the path is dynamic, filled with highs and lows and that each stage adds to the fabric of our overall well-being is important.

Through my journey, I came to understand that the actual meaning of fitness is not just about physical change, but also about a change in mindset and way of life.

Long-Term Wellness and Health

Long-term health and wellness are noble and arduous goals to pursue. It goes beyond the ebb and flow of fads, fashions, and quick fixes. It represents a constant dedication to the health of our bodies, brains, and spirits. We examine the value of long-term health and wellness in this last chapter, recognizing it as a holistic endeavor that includes physical vitality, mental toughness, emotional balance, and a life filled with meaning.

The essence of our physical well-being is at the center of long-term health and wellness. It is a recognition that our bodies are complex ecosystems that require care and respect rather than just being empty vessels. This care starts with nutrition, a deliberate and informed decision about the foods we eat. Food is not only a source of nutrition but also the building block of good health. It requires finding balance, being aware of our decisions, and providing our bodies with the critical nutrition they need. It involves adopting healthy food choices that encourage vitality and longevity while enjoying pleasures that make you happy without doing any harm.

Regular exercise is a further component of physical well-being. Moving our bodies is a lifelong commitment, not a temporary duty. Exercise includes a wide range of activities, from cardiovascular workouts to strengthening our muscles and maintaining our functional mobility. It is an awareness that exercise benefits one's health and raises the quality of life rather than only being for aesthetic purposes. It's about recognizing our bodies' ongoing capacity to change, develop, and flourish when we provide them with movement.

The third pillar of physical well-being is getting enough rest and recovering. Sleep, which is frequently overlooked in terms of its importance, is an essential element that supports both physical and cognitive activities. It serves as a reminder that finding time to unwind and refresh is not only necessary but also desirable. It involves giving our bodies and minds the attention they need to be renewed because they are our greatest resources as we travel through life.

However, the road to long-term fitness and health goes beyond the body. It also includes mental and emotional health. A healthy mind serves as our compass as we navigate the joys and difficulties of life. Resilience, emotional intelligence, and stress management abilities are all developed as a result. It is a recognition that life's vicissitudes are a part of the human experience and that how we handle them has a significant impact on how well we are able to function in general.

In order to maintain mental well-being and emotional health, it is crucial to cultivate loving relationships, practice self-compassion, and ask for help when necessary. Also, it is a recognition of the power of vulnerability and the importance of genuine connections to our pleasure. It serves as a reminder that fostering emotional connections enriches our lives and strengthens our feeling of community.

Long-term health and wellness are goals that must be pursued holistically and are woven into the fabric of our lives. It acknowledges the role that our daily decisions and routines have in determining our long-term well-being. As part of an all-encompassing strategy, mindfulness is accepted as a technique for developing self-awareness and intentionality. It involves being in the moment and making decisions that are consistent with our values and objectives.

In addition, long-term wellness values the development of interests, passions, and creativity. These activities promote happiness and allow for self-expression, which adds to our overall sense of contentment.

It takes a community to achieve long-term health and fitness. It thrives in the protection of caring communities and thanks to a higher purpose than personal happiness. Engagement in the community, whether it is through friendships, service projects, or mentorship, improves our lives and strengthens our sense of belonging. A sense of direction and motivation is provided by a sense of purpose, which might come from one's work, personal objectives, or efforts to further the common good. It serves as a reminder that our well-being is entwined with that of others and the environment.

Conclusion

We are not at the end of this investigation into long-term health and wellness; rather, we are at the beginning of an endless odyssey. Every action we take, decision we make, and experience we have on this path is infused with the profound knowledge that our health is a treasure, a duty, and a gift we provide to the rest of the world and ourselves.

We've explored the many facets of wellness and come to understand that it includes not just the health of our physical bodies but also the resiliency of our brains, the harmony of our emotions, and the balance of our lifestyles. Our physical health, mental stamina, emotional intelligence, and the enduring search for meaning and connection are intricately woven together in one holistic tapestry.

We have discovered the enduring principles that direct us on this trip in the chapters of this book. We now understand that a healthy diet is the foundation of our physical vitality, that engaging in regular exercise requires a lifetime commitment, and that adequate rest and recuperation are essential elements of our overall well-being.

Let us begin this endless voyage as we stand at this doorway with hearts full of appreciation and intention. Let's make decisions that demonstrate our dedication to well-being in order to respect the knowledge we have received from these pages. Let's treasure each breath, each conversation, and each moment as an opportunity to take care of our well-being.

Let's keep in mind as we go that the goal of this expedition is to embrace the route rather than the final destination. Living fully means embracing each day as a chance to enhance our well-being and improve the well-being of others as well as global well-being.

May our quest for long-term health and wellness be a brilliant thread that adds beauty, vibrancy, and significance to the rich fabric of our lives in the great tapestry of existence.